If I'm DEAD and you are making my arrangements, START HERE
(and hopefully I have already filled in the pages!)

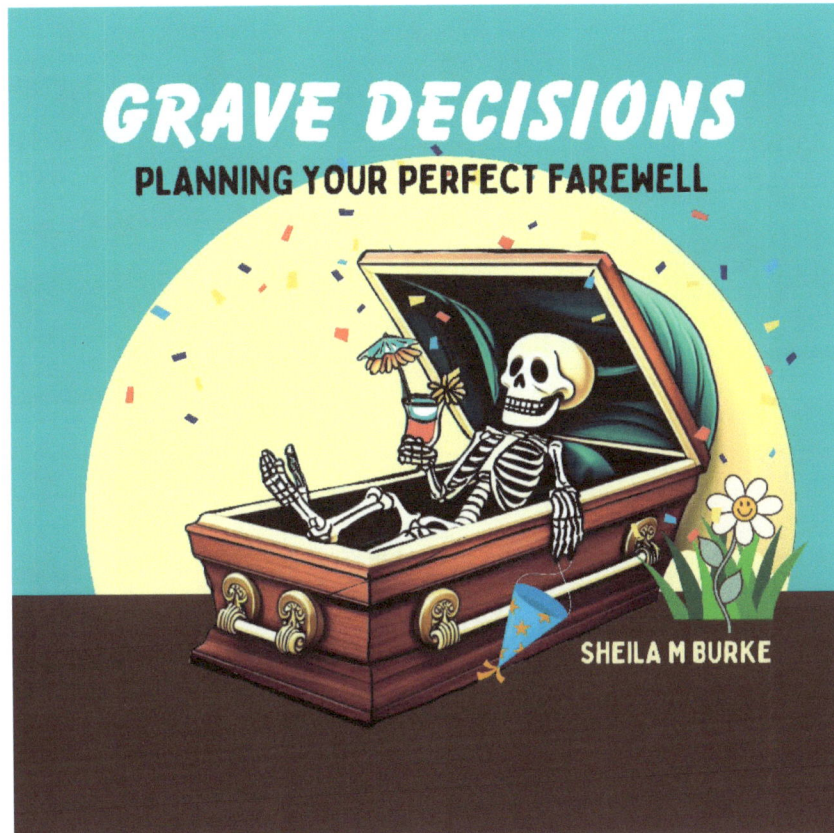

GRAVE DECISIONS
PLANNING YOUR PERFECT FAREWELL

SHEILA M BURKE

ISBN: 979-8-9859214-5-8

OmSweetOm Publishing

Cleveland, OH 44131

Author photo by Rachel Barrett

Cover design by Sheila Burke

Disclaimer

The information provided in this book is for general informational purposes only and is not intended to serve as legal advice. While efforts have been made to ensure accuracy, laws and regulations regarding end-of-life planning and related topics vary by jurisdiction and may change over time. Readers are encouraged to consult with qualified legal, medical, or financial professionals for advice tailored to their specific circumstances. The author and publisher disclaim any liability for decisions made based on the information provided in this book.

TABLE OF CONTENTS

Well, it's YOUR Funeral

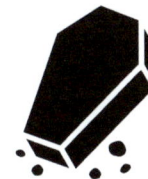

Exploring the Afterlife's Real Estate Market: A Guide to Burial Options

Planning your funeral? Congratulations—you're ahead of the curve! While most people avoid thinking about death, you've decided to embrace it with humor and flair. Choosing your final resting place is no small feat, but don't worry; this guide is here to help. Let's dive into the fabulous (and occasionally bizarre) world of burial options.

Traditional Burial

The OG of burials. You get a coffin, a plot in a cemetery, and a headstone where loved ones can leave flowers and awkwardly avoid stepping on someone else's grave. It's a timeless choice, but it does come with decisions: mahogany or pine? Satin lining or something more eco-friendly? How about the extras—do you want that fancy waterproof vault, or are you keeping it simple?

Then there's the cemetery plot. It's like prime real estate—location, location, location! Do you prefer a scenic spot under a peaceful oak tree, a sunny patch near the edge, or something close to the main gate for easy drive-by visits? And let's not forget the neighbors—you might end up between "Beloved Grandma Edith" and "Here Lies Joe, Gone Too Soon But Not Soon Enough (Just Kidding)."

Plus, think about the headstone—classic marble, polished granite, or something quirky like a bench so visitors can sit and chat with you? The possibilities are endless. If you're feeling fancy, maybe throw in a custom epitaph like, "Told You I Was Sick" or "Living the Quiet Life Now." Your final resting place deserves personality!

Cremation

Why take up space when you can become stardust (or at least a fine powder)? Cremation offers flexibility: your cremains (ashes) can be scattered in a beloved location, stored in an urn, or even transformed into jewelry. That's right—you can become a diamond. Talk about leaving a legacy! Bonus points if you request something unique, like having your ashes launched into space or mixed into fireworks. Who wouldn't want their final send-off to go out with a bang?

Green Burial

For the eco-conscious soul, green burial skips the embalming chemicals and fancy caskets. You're buried directly in the earth, wrapped in a biodegradable shroud, or placed in a simple, untreated wooden box. Essentially, you're giving back to Mother Nature—becoming a literal tree hugger as your body nourishes the soil. If you've spent your life recycling, why stop at death?

Burial at Sea

Cue the theme from *Titanic* and set sail into eternity. Burial at sea is perfect for those who love the ocean. It's not as simple as dropping your ashes overboard; there are regulations to follow. Whether you choose cremated remains or a full-body burial (in a weighted, biodegradable shroud, of course), this option promises a watery grave with a view. Just make sure you're okay with sharing your final resting place with schools of fish.

Alkaline Hydrolysis (AKA Water Cremation)

The cutting-edge cousin of cremation involves dissolving your body in a water-based solution. Think of it as a gentle, eco-friendly way to return to nature. The remaining liquid is safe for disposal (yes, down the drain) while the bone fragments can be turned into ashes for your loved ones. Science meets sentimentality in this futuristic farewell.

Space Burial

For the dreamers and sci-fi fans, a space burial lets you escape Earth's gravitational pull for good. A small portion of your ashes is launched into orbit or beyond. Prices vary depending on how far you want to go—low Earth orbit is more budget-friendly, while a trip to the Moon will cost a little more. But hey, how many people can say, "I'm spending eternity among the stars"?

Mummification

Want to go full ancient Egyptian? Mummification is still an option. There's a company in the U.S. that will embalm and wrap you like a pharaoh, ensuring your body stays intact for centuries. This one's perfect if you want future archaeologists to marvel at your fabulous taste in burial attire.

Human Composting

Officially called natural organic reduction, this method turns your body into nutrient-rich soil. Over a few weeks, you'll transform into compost that your loved ones can use to plant a tree or grow a garden. It's poetic, really—you spend your whole life feeding the world, and now you're helping feed the earth.

Cryonics

For those who aren't quite ready to say goodbye, cryonics offers the chance to be frozen in liquid nitrogen. The idea is that someday when science catches up, you'll be revived and ready to rejoin society. Of course, there's no guarantee this will work, but it's a great conversation starter for the future scientists who thaw you out.

Eco Burial Pods

Want to become a tree? Burial pods take green burial to the next level. Your body is placed in a biodegradable pod along with the seed of your choice. As you decompose, you nourish the tree, essentially becoming part of it. Apple tree? Oak? Cherry blossom? Choose your legacy wisely—people might be eating pies made from your nutrients one day.

Novelty Burials

For the ultimate personalization, consider unique burial options. Have your ashes pressed into a vinyl record, mixed into tattoo ink, or encased in a coral reef structure. Your final resting place can reflect your hobbies, passions, or even your sense of humor. Who wouldn't want to spend eternity as part of a reef, helping Nemo find his way home?

Fill in: What to do with my body

Final Thoughts

Choosing your burial method is the ultimate act of self-expression. Whether you go traditional or quirky, remember that this is *your* journey into the great beyond. So why not have some fun with it? After all, death is the one thing we all have in common—might as well make it memorable.

From Dust to Delight: Fun Things to Do with Your Cremains

1. The Scenic Scatter
The classic scattering of ashes is beautiful, but why not spice it up? Tell your family to scatter you somewhere truly wild—off a roller coaster, from a hot air balloon, or during halftime at a sporting event. Just be sure to leave behind detailed instructions and maybe bail money, depending on the location.

2. Become Bling
Yes, you can become a diamond, but why stop there? Suggest being turned into a whole jewelry line. Picture it: Cousin Karen wearing "Aunt Sue" earrings at Christmas dinner, trying to act normal. Let your family drip in your brilliance while you remain the ultimate ice queen (or king).

3. Fireworks Finale
It's hard to cry when Grandma's ashes are exploding into a glittering red, white, and blue spectacle. Insist on a full pyrotechnic show with a synchronized soundtrack. And don't hold back—this is your last party. Bonus points if you write your will in sparkler font.

4. Get Shot Into Space
Nothing says, "I've always been out of this world" like becoming intergalactic dust. Let your ashes boldly go where no one has gone before—or at least into low Earth orbit. Be sure to demand your family play *Also Sprach Zarathustra* (the *2001: A Space Odyssey* theme) as the rocket takes off.

5. Memorial Jewelry (Beyond Diamonds)
Why stick to just diamonds when there's an entire jewelry box of possibilities? Your ashes can be incorporated into glass beads, pendants, lockets, or even fused with metals to create one-of-a-kind rings and necklaces. It's a stylish way for loved ones to carry you close, literally turning grief into wearable art. Plus, you'll always be part of someone's outfit of the day.

6. Get Artsy
Why settle for a tasteful painting when you can star in an avant-garde masterpiece? Tell your family to commission a self-portrait where the artist incorporates your ashes and just enough glitter to make people *really uncomfortable*. Bonus: future generations can argue over whether it's creepy or cool.

7. Tattoo You

For the ultimate permanent mark, your ashes can be mixed into tattoo ink and used to create meaningful (or quirky) tattoos for your loved ones. You'll be literally under your loved one's skin, and isn't that what family is all about? Suggest something hilarious, like "This tattoo is dead serious" or "Grandma's here—don't mess up." Watch as your family debates whether it's genius or a terrible idea, just like every other family decision. Whether it's a delicate design like your handwriting or something funnier—like your face with the words "I told you I'd haunt you"—you'll live on in their skin. It's a mix of legacy and modern art, plus a great conversation starter.

8. Reef Revival

Becoming part of a coral reef sounds peaceful—until you realize a parrotfish might nibble on you. Still, imagine your family scuba-diving down to visit you, only to find a clownfish has taken up residence. "Grandpa, is that you?"

9. Hourglass of Eternity

Not only is this a poetic reminder of life's fleeting nature, but it's also wildly practical. Tell your family to use you during games of Pictionary, ensuring you'll still be the one keeping them all on time. You'll forever be at game night—whether you liked game night or not!

10. Vinyl Record Vibes

Why not make music part of your afterlife if music was your jam? Your ashes can be pressed into a vinyl record with grooves that play your favorite songs, voice recordings, or even quirky soundbites ("Put me down!"). Your loved ones can rock out or reminisce to the literal soundtrack of your life. It's the ultimate mixtape, just on a slightly more eternal scale.

11. Shot Glass Shenanigans

Turn your ashes into shot glasses and be the life of every party, one drink at a time. Insist they toast with your favorite drink and a chant of, "One for the road, Grandpa!" Also, maybe engrave "Bottoms up!" on the base for an extra laugh.

12. Action Figure Encore

Imagine your family dusting off your custom action figure years later, saying, "Remember when Grandpa thought this was a good idea?" Add accessories like a cape, tiny golf clubs, or even a removable toupee.

13. Bowling Ball Brilliance

Roll into eternity with style! Insist on being turned into a custom bowling ball, complete with your name etched on the side. Bonus points if your family organizes an annual memorial bowling tournament called "The Last Roll."

14. Ash-Infused Concrete

You could become part of a park bench, but why stop there? Tell your family to mix your ashes into concrete for a DIY backyard barbecue pit or even a garden statue that looks suspiciously like you.

15. Ashes to Ammo

If you've always been a straight shooter, why not keep that energy going? Have your ashes loaded into shotgun shells or rifle cartridges so your family can take you on one last hunting trip or to the skeet range. It's the ultimate way to go out with a bang—just make sure they don't aim at anything awkward, like the family cabin or Dad's old fishing hat.

16. Eternal Snow Globe

Shake things up—literally. Turn yourself into a snow globe, but make it seasonal. Suggest a "Halloween Grandma" theme with a tiny witch figure inside. That way, you'll always be a hit during spooky season.

17. Coffee Mug Companion

There's nothing cozier than starting your day with "a piece of Dad." Have your ashes incorporated into ceramic mugs with inspirational quotes like, "You've still got time... but not much."

18. Frisbee Forever

Stay in the game by becoming a custom Frisbee. Whether it's the dog fetching you or the grandkids flinging you across the park, you'll ensure that no one ever forgets who has the best throw in the family.

19. Vinyl Decal Memorial

Be the bumper sticker that lives on forever. Whether it's on your grandkid's laptop or stuck to the family RV, suggest something memorable like, "If you can read this, I'm haunting you."

20. A Time Capsule Surprise

Why just leave a will when you can leave a mystery? Why settle for fading into obscurity when you can rise from the ground like a Netflix mystery series? Pack your ashes into a time capsule with some cryptic notes, bizarre trinkets, and maybe a fake treasure map for good measure. Bury it in the backyard or some remote location, and let future generations unearth you like an ancient pharaoh—minus the curse (or with one if you're feeling spicy). Perfect for keeping your descendants on their toes and wondering, *"Was Great-Grandma always this extra?"*

21. Memorial Kite
Soar into the sky one last time. Your ashes can be part of a custom kite that the family flies every windy day. Just hope they don't lose you to a powerline.

22. Ashes to Soap
Nothing says "clean family values" like turning yourself into a set of soap bars. Insist on a scent that'll really make an impression, like lavender... or bacon.

23. Poker Chip Pal
You always had a poker face—now you'll be the face of the poker game. Your family can bring you to Vegas, stacking you high for the ultimate all-in bet. Don't bluff too hard, though; your game might be dead, but your reputation isn't.

24. Balloon Release (But Make It You)
Fill biodegradable balloons with your ashes, then watch as your family releases them into the sky. Just make sure they have a backup plan in case the wind sends you into a neighbor's pool party.

25. Message in a Bottle
Put your ashes and a cryptic note in a bottle and let the tide take you. Whoever finds it will either think you're a long-lost pirate or a very dedicated prankster.

26. Puppet Encore
Who wouldn't want to star in one last puppet show? Turn your ashes into part of a marionette, and let your family recreate your best moments at birthdays, weddings, or *very* awkward funerals.

27. Become Part of a Garden Gnome
"Eternal resting gnome" has a nice ring to it. Turn yourself into a backyard statue, but make it hilarious—like a gnome mooning the neighbor's yard. Now you'll have the best seat for every family barbecue.

28. Custom Candles
Light up the room, literally. Insist your family mix your ashes into candles and use them only for power outages or romantic dinners. Scent idea: "Smells Like Grandpa's Garage."

Final Thoughts

Your ashes deserve to be as unique and hilarious as your life was. So dream big, lean into the absurd, and leave your family with stories they'll never stop laughing about—or questioning. After all, why rest in peace when you can rest in *pieces* of pure comedy?

Fill in: what to do with my cremains

PICK A THEME!

Funerals, Your Way:
Traditions, Themes, and Everything in Between

Planning your own funeral might sound grim, but let's face it: this is your *last* chance to throw a party. So, why not make it one to remember? Whether you lean toward classic traditions or prefer to turn your final farewell into an event for the ages, there's no wrong way to say goodbye—except maybe leaving it all to Cousin Bob, who once tried to serve potato salad *without* mayo.

The TRADITIONAL FUNERAL CUSTOMS Box

If you're a fan of time-honored traditions, start here.

Think back to your family's customs or your religious preferences. Do you envision hymns and eulogies in a peaceful chapel? A procession to a favorite burial site? Or maybe a good old-fashioned wake with enough casseroles to feed a small army?

Here's where you write down the details. Be as specific as you want:

- Favorite prayers, hymns, or readings.
- Special attire for the guests (*yes, kilts count!*).
- Anything you'd *never* want, like Aunt Edna's accordion solo making a comeback.

Themed Funerals: Because Why Should Weddings Have All the Fun?

If traditional isn't your style, why not pick a theme? Yes, a *theme*. Your funeral can reflect your passions, hobbies, or that one phase where you were really into pirate reenactments.

Here are some ideas to get you started:

- **For the Sports Enthusiast:** A tailgate funeral, complete with stadium snacks, jerseys, and guests doing the wave as your casket takes its final lap. Bonus points for halftime highlights of your life on a big screen.
- **For the Bookworm:** A literary-themed funeral where everyone comes dressed as their favorite character. Your eulogy? Delivered in the style of Shakespeare, of course. "Alas, poor [Your Name]— we knew them well!"
- **For the Adventurer:** A National Park-themed service where your ashes (or a replica) are displayed in a miniature tent, surrounded by pine-scented candles and trail mix. Include a slideshow of your travels and send guests home with maps to your favorite hikes.
- **For the Foodie:** A "Last Supper" banquet featuring your favorite dishes. Each course could represent a milestone in your life. Appetizer: Birth. Entrée: Career. Dessert: "Don't Cry for Me, I'm With the Cheesecake Now."
- **For the Jokester:** A comedy club-themed service. Have a lineup of friends and family tell funny stories about you. Leave behind cue cards for one-liners like, "I told you I wasn't feeling great!"

Can't Decide? Go for Both!

Why limit yourself to one style when you can combine them? Start with a traditional service, and end with a themed afterparty. Maybe it's a solemn church ceremony, followed by a Star Trek-themed reception with a Klingon officiant yelling, *"Today is a good day to die!"*

Or vice versa: kick things off with a costume party, and let everyone wind down with a quiet candlelit vigil. It's your funeral—do what feels right (*and slightly fabulous*).

- **Jazzed-Up Serenity:** Begin with a traditional funeral service complete with hymns, candles, and heartfelt prayers, but follow it up with a New Orleans-style jazz procession. Picture it: a brass band leading your loved ones in a parade, transitioning from somber tunes to upbeat melodies as they march to your final resting place. Mourning and celebrating all in one? *Chef's kiss.*
- **Classic Yet Campy:** Start with a dignified graveside service featuring floral arrangements and a touching eulogy. Then surprise everyone with a costume-themed potluck reception where guests

dress up as historical figures from your favorite era. Nothing says "honoring a life well-lived" like seeing Uncle Joe dressed as Benjamin Franklin while eating deviled eggs.

- **Quiet Reflection to Karaoke Perfection:** Begin with a serene memorial service, complete with a moment of silence, touching tributes, and maybe some tear-jerking harp music. Then crank up the vibes at the reception with a full-blown karaoke party where everyone sings your favorite tunes. Bonus points if the playlist includes *"Stayin' Alive"* and *"My Way"*—because irony is the ultimate crowd-pleaser.

The Final Word

Whether you're jotting down sacred traditions or envisioning a disco ball and karaoke machine at your wake, the key is this: Make it *you*. Your life was one-of-a-kind, and your funeral should be, too. So grab that pen and start planning—because if anyone deserves to have the last laugh (or hymn), it's you.

Alright, Let's Plan That Party!

Time to figure out your grand finale. Do you want a *funeral*—the classic option with your body (or ashes) taking center stage? Or maybe a *memorial service*—basically the same vibe, but you've already exited stage left. Then there's the wild card: a *celebration of life*. Think less tears, more laughs, and possibly a chocolate fountain.

Here's the big question: If you go with a celebration of life, should it happen immediately after your departure or give people a bit of time to miss you first? Circle one below:

- Funeral
- Memorial Service
- Celebration of Life (ASAP)
- Celebration of Life (After Everyone Stops Ugly Crying)
- OR... I don't want anything at all

No pressure, but remember—this is your last party, so make it count!

Who Says Funerals Can't Have a Treat Bag?

If you're skipping the traditional religious route, congrats—you've got way more options! First, pick your venue: a funeral home, your favorite hiking trail, or maybe that dive bar where everyone knows your order, or a scenic beachside ceremony. And speaking of parties—every good one has party favors or treat bags, right? Why not work that into your funeral? A little something for the road, like a tiny jar of your favorite candy, a mini bottle of whiskey, or a note saying, *"Thanks for coming! See you in the afterlife!"*

Party favors: not just for kids' birthdays anymore.

Our family honored our fisherman brother-in-law with a bowl of bobbers—simple, sentimental, and pocket-sized. We celebrated my husband, a golfer, by offering guests golf tees, perfect for remembering all those afternoons spent on the green. Need more inspiration? Try packets of flower seeds for the gardener, mini chocolate bars for the sweet tooth in your life, or even a bowl of your loved one's favorite snacks (because who wouldn't want to be remembered over a bag of hot Cheetos?). For nature lovers, you could go big with small sapling trees, or keep it artsy with hand-painted rocks.

The key is to make it personal. Whether guests leave with a tiny keepsake or just a good laugh, these thoughtful touches ensure they'll remember your celebration—not just the awkward hug from Aunt Edna.

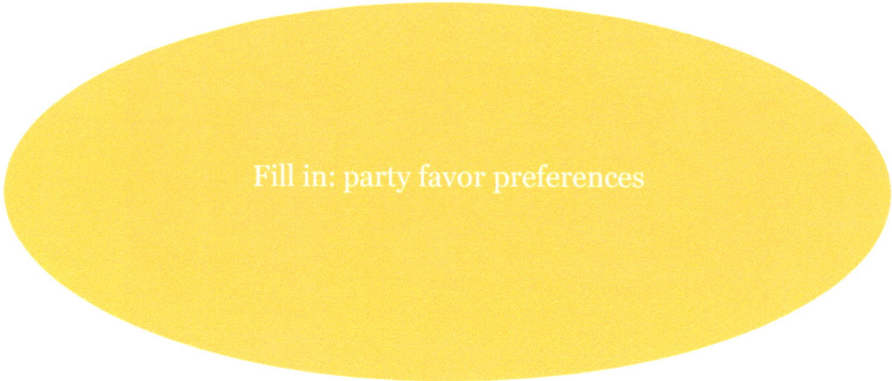

Fill in: party favor preferences

PRE-PLANNED ARRANGEMENTS

I DO   I DO NOT   have any arrangements currently pre-paid. If yes, what and where

_____

_____

_____

14

Do you want to be buried with any specific or special items?

Any Special Items for the Afterlife? Let's Talk Grave Swag.

So, what's going in the casket with you? Some people opt for sentimental keepsakes—like Grandma's rosary or that lucky rabbit's foot you swear got you through high school algebra. Others go for something more *practical,* like a flashlight (just in case) or a Snickers (because you're not you when you're hungry).

Want to really keep it interesting? Toss in something to confuse future archaeologists—like a remote control, a signed headshot of Nicolas Cage, or a note that says, *"You're next."*

It's your call! Whether it's a love letter, a family heirloom, or that pair of socks you never let anyone borrow, make sure your grave goods are as unique as you. After all, you can't take it with you unless you literally do.

Let's Play Dress up!

Pick your own outfit (Don't be caught dead in something you don't like.)

Fill in your general style or a specific outfit

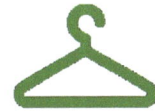

Style is a way to say who you are **Without** having to speak. -Rachel Zoe

THINGS TO THINK ABOUT:
OBITUARY AND LEGACY.

Writing Your Own Obituary: The Most Fun You'll Ever Have Planning to Be Dead

Let's Get Serious for a Second

Writing your own obituary or legacy statement is like creating your highlight reel. You get to frame your story the way you want it told, ensuring no one leaves out the important stuff (*like that time you finally beat Cousin Todd at Scrabble*). It's a chance to reflect on your life, celebrate your wins, and decide what really matters.

And let's face it, the benefits are huge:

- **You Control the Narrative**: No one's going to gloss over your epic karaoke championship win or your legendary Thanksgiving stuffing recipe.
- **No Awkward Guesswork**: Your family won't have to squabble over whether you were 5'8" or 5'10" (*for the record, you were always 5'10" in heels*).
- **A Legacy That Feels Like *You***: Your story, your voice, your vibe. Whether you want it heartfelt, hilarious, or deeply poetic, you're in charge.

Now, Let's Make It Fun!

Why let someone else write your send-off when you can do it yourself—better, funnier, and way more accurate? Think of it as your final creative project, with no pesky deadlines (well, except *that* one).

Here's how to have a blast with it:

- **Brag Shamelessly**: Write like no one's going to fact-check. "They climbed Everest twice, invented the cheese grater, and once saved a kitten from a burning building."
- **Add Humor**: "They leave behind a loving family, three suspiciously well-fed cats, and an impressive collection of half-finished DIY projects."
- **Drop Some Wisdom**: Share your life's greatest lesson: "Always bet on yourself. And never trust a fart past 50."
- **Go Out with a Bang**: Sign off with something unforgettable, like "See you in the great buffet in the sky—save me a seat by the desserts."

Why it's Totally Worth It

Writing your own obituary isn't morbid—it's liberating. It's your chance to tell your story your way, to have the last laugh (literally), and to leave your loved ones with something that's 100% *you*. Plus, let's be honest, it's way more fun than organizing the junk drawer or watching reruns of *Wheel of Fortune*.

So grab a pen, pour a drink, and get started. You've got a legacy to craft—and this time, you really can write your own ending.

If you are struggling to write your own, at least give your loved ones some facts about yourself so that someone else can write a proper obituary for you. Answers to these questions should give them the information they need to complete an obit.

What are your accomplishments or achievements?

What are your hobbies and interests?

Is there anything you want to be sure of is included in your obituary?

Where have you lived during your life? Were you a traveler?

What are your favorite things, places, or jobs?

What is your education?

Did you serve in the military? Years, rank, location

What were your professions during your life?

Which quality or character trait of yours would you most like to be passed down as your legacy?

Are there certain possessions that you would like specific people to receive when you die?

Would you like to have something done in remembrance of you, for example, a memorial tree, bench, or garden?

How would you like your birthday, or your death day remembered?

How do you want to be remembered? Think about it and pick 3-5 things you want people to remember you for.

These are a few of my **~favorite things~**

Knowing a person's favorite things plays a beneficial role in planning a funeral, celebration, or writing a eulogy. Fill in what you can. Come back later to the answers you leave blank. (If you are still alive.)

3 favorite bands/groups/singers

_____

_____

_____

Song

_____

_____

Movie

_____

Book

_____

3 Favorite Flowers

_____

_____

3 Favorite Colors

_____

_____

Favorite Beer

_____

Wine

_____

Coffee flavor

_____

Tea flavor or brand

_____

TV Show

_____

Favorite F.R.I.E.N.D.S Character

_____

Favorite Gilligan's Island Character

_____

Favorite Simpson's Character

_____

Holiday_____

Charity_____

Places to travel

_____

Flavor of Ice Cream

_____

Pizza Topping(s)

_____

Food

_____

Drink

_____

Dessert

_____

Animal or bird

_____

Sport

_____

Sports Team

_____

_____

_____

Pastime

_____

_____

_____

Favorite Quotes:

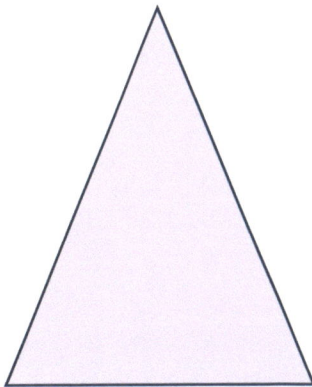

Funeral and Remembrance Ideas~

Funerals and celebrations of life are highly customizable. Whether you are planning your funeral, or a loved one's, here are some ideas to make it memorable.

👕 Creating a Dress Code for Your Funeral: Because Who Says You Can't Look Fabulous While Departing?

Why let your funeral be just another somber gathering in dull black suits? Nope! This is your last hurrah, and you're in charge of the dress code. Think of it as your final party—only this time, the theme is "Make It Memorable!" So go ahead and get creative!

Here's the deal:

You could put out a simple request: "Anything but black!" Just imagine the scene: your friends and family rocking bright Hawaiian shirts, neon colors, or even their favorite sports team jerseys. It's a celebration of your life, after all, and who doesn't want to remember you while looking like a beach party?

Fun Dress Code Ideas:

1. **Hawaiian Paradise:** "Come in your best Hawaiian attire—grass skirts, leis, and flip-flops encouraged. Bonus points for grass skirts that make people wonder if they're at a funeral or a luau!"
2. **Team Spirit:** "Wear your favorite sports team gear. Imagine a sea of jerseys—everyone fighting over who gets to eulogize you first based on the teams' records. It's a great way to get your family to finally put their sports rivalries aside (at least for one day)."
3. **Color Explosion:** "Please dress in your favorite color—let's create a rainbow! And remember, if someone shows up in black, they'll have to sing 'Somewhere over the Rainbow' on stage."
4. **Costume Party:** "Show up as your favorite movie character or historical figure. Just imagine Uncle Bob arriving as a pirate while Aunt Judy tries to channel Cleopatra. It's going to be the most chaotic, hilarious funeral ever!"
5. **Formal and Funky:** "Wear your best formal attire—tuxedos, ball gowns, and all—but make it funky. Think sequins, feather boas, and hats that could double as small umbrellas. Why blend in when you can stand out in style?"

The Final Touch:

As guests arrive, hand out quirky accessories: glow sticks, oversized sunglasses, or even a fun hat to complete the look. Think of it as a party favor that says, "I may be gone, but I'm here to ensure you have the best time while you mourn me!"

So go ahead and make those fashion requests! You're the host of this ultimate event, so let your friends know that this isn't just a farewell; it's a celebration of life, laughter, and the ridiculousness of it all. After all, if you can't rock a flower crown at your own funeral, when can you?

WHAT WOULD YOU LIKE TO HAVE AS A DRESS CODE FOR YOUR FUNERAL?

_____

_____

_____

_____

Memory Table

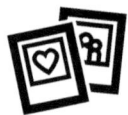

The Ultimate Tribute to Your Awesomeness!

Whether you're going the traditional route with a body on display or just bringing your cremains along for the ride, one thing's for sure: you need a memory table. This is the spot where your friends and family can gather to reminisce about all the wonderful (and slightly ridiculous) moments of your life.

So, what goes on this magical table of memories? It's not just about the photos—though feel free to include that one where you were wearing your dad's old glasses and pretending to be a pirate. You should also toss in anything that represents your fabulous self:

- **Favorite Books**: Those dog-eared novels you claimed you'd reread but never got around to. Bonus points if they're so dusty that even the Grim Reaper sneezes!
- **Memorabilia**: That hideous mug you won for "Employee of the Month" (which you may have had to share with your cat). Maybe some funky collectibles, like that singing fish plaque that no one knows how you acquired.

- **Hobby Highlights**: A mini display of your hobbies—be it your knitting projects (sorry, Aunt Sue), your model train collection that's taken over the living room, or the half-finished jigsaw puzzle that was clearly never meant to be solved.
- **Sports Fanaticism**: Have your favorite team's memorabilia on display—just remember to include a note that says, *"Yes, they've won a championship! No, you can't blame me for the losing seasons."*

And don't forget to throw in a few quirky items that reflect your personality. Maybe a rubber chicken, a kazoo, or that "World's Okayest Human" mug you insisted was a great gift.

Ultimately, the memory table should scream, *"This was me, and I was fabulous!"* It's the perfect way to spark stories, share laughs, and keep the memories alive—while secretly judging everyone for not dressing as fabulously as you requested! So set up that table with pride and watch your loved ones gather around, swapping tales and wondering how they'll ever top your legendary life.

WHAT WOULD YOU LIKE ON YOUR MEMORY TABLE?

_____

_____

_____

_____

Be creative with food and drink 🍩

Taste and Smell: The Secret Weapon of Memory Lane

Let's be real: one of the best ways to trigger a memory is through taste and scent. Seriously, nothing brings back those warm, fuzzy feelings like a whiff of Grandma's secret sauce or the taste of that questionable casserole Aunt Mildred swears is "the family recipe" (but you're pretty sure came from a can).

So, what's the decedent's favorite food? It's time to share those culinary delights! Print out their prized recipes and let visitors take home a little taste of nostalgia. You can include them in the funeral program, slap them on the back of the funeral home card, or showcase them on the memory table for everyone to fight over. Imagine the scene: family members grabbing recipes, hoping to recreate that one dish that had everyone fighting for seconds—or at least keep the family tradition alive of no one actually following the recipe correctly. "Oh, Grandma's famous lasagna? You mean the one that requires 37 secret ingredients and a sprinkle of love that's always mysteriously missing?"

Plus, handing out recipes is a great way to spark conversations, like, "Remember when Cousin Bob tried to make this and ended up setting the kitchen on fire? Good times!" So, print those recipes loud and proud! After all, nothing says *"I'm still here in spirit"* like making everyone enjoy your cooking (or at least give them a good laugh). Just be sure to include a disclaimer: *"Culinary successes not guaranteed; may cause food comas or spontaneous family gatherings."*

If serving food at the funeral/celebration, consider having a table that includes the deceased favorite(s):

_____
_____
_____
_____
_____
_____
_____

Encourage visitors to share, participate, and remember together

Invite Friends and Family to Share a Memory: The Ultimate Roast or Toast!

Gather your friends and family and let them know it's time to share their best memories, stories, or messages about you. This isn't just a sentimental moment; it's a chance for them to take the mic and unleash their inner comedian (or emotional poet). Who knows, maybe Uncle Larry will finally confess to that embarrassing incident at the family reunion, or Aunt Joan will reveal how you once tried to impress her with your "amazing" dance moves that were more "awkward giraffe" than "smooth operator."

Encouraging everyone to share their favorite tales is a beautiful way to reflect on your life, and trust me, these stories will become family legends. Years down the line, they'll be reminiscing about that time you dressed as a pirate for Halloween and forgot to take off your eye patch during Thanksgiving dinner. You'll be remembered not just for the life you lived but for the laughs you brought!

So, hand out some mic time, set up a comfy chair, and let the storytelling begin. It's the perfect blend of humor and heartfelt reflection, ensuring that your legacy lives on in laughter and love. After all, life is too short to be serious all the time—except when it comes to eating the last piece of cake, of course. Alternatively, you could set up a table and have people write their memories and put the papers into a basket to read later.

Lights, Camera, Legacy!

Why let your life be summarized in a boring obituary when you can go *full Hollywood*? Instead, create a slideshow or video that showcases your greatest hits (and maybe a few bloopers). Here's how to turn your life into a blockbuster—or at least a memorable photo montage:

Option 1: The Slideshow Spectacular
Gather your best photos—baby you rocking a diaper, teenage you rocking questionable 90s fashion, and grown-up you rocking...well, life. Add captions that capture the essence of each moment, like:

- *"First steps (and first face plant)."*
- *"That time I thought bangs were a good idea."*
- *"The love of my life and partner in crime, (your spouse, partner, etc)—my forever co-star."*

Then, set it all to music. Go for a soundtrack that screams YOU, whether it's "Eye of the Tiger" for the action-packed moments or a tearjerker ballad for the sentimental bits. Bonus points if you throw in some comic relief slides, like "What Not to Wear: 2003 Edition."

Option 2: The Feature Film

Why stop at photos? Create a video and narrate it like the epic journey it is. Sprinkle in some one-liners:

- *"This is the exact moment I realized heels and hiking don't mix."*
- *"Here's the lasagna I burned the night I tried to impress the in-laws."*
- *"This is me laughing so hard I cried because life was ridiculous—and also amazing."*

Not tech-savvy? Recruit the family tech guru. Bribe them with pizza, and voila—you've got a Spielberg in the making.

Option 3: Memory Board Magic

For a low-tech but equally fabulous option, create a memory board filled with photos, ticket stubs, postcards, and other mementos. Add captions or funny commentary to each piece:

- That blurry photo from the road trip? Label it *"Yes, that's my thumb covering the Grand Canyon."*
- A postcard from Spain? Write, *"The week I learned siesta culture was made for me."*

Stick it all on a giant board, and you've got an exhibit-worthy piece of art. Put it up at your celebration of life or family gatherings—it's bound to spark laughter, tears, and a few *"I can't believe you saved this!"* moments.

So go ahead—get creative! Whether it's a slideshow, a short film, or a scrapbook masterpiece, this is your chance to tell your story your way. After all, who better to narrate your life than the person who lived it?

Giveaway/gifting ideas

The Ultimate Posthumous Giveaway: Clearing Out the Closet!

We've already tackled the fabulous party favors for your funeral, but why stop there? Consider gifting away personal items, too! Think of it as your final chance to host a "take what you want" party—without the awkward chit-chat or risk of Aunt Edna spilling her punch all over your favorite rug.

Now, a little disclaimer: it's best to give yourself some time before you start handing things out. You don't want to be the person giving away Grandma's favorite porcelain cat collection right after she's gone (let's save that for the family reunion drama later).

So, what's in your treasure trove? Did the deceased have a mountain of shirts that could outfit a small army? A collection of hats that rival a milliner's? Or maybe a stack of books so tall it could be a fire hazard? It's time to turn that clutter into cherished mementos!

Picture it: loved ones eagerly picking through the goods, exclaiming things like, "I always wanted to borrow this shirt!" or "Who knew Uncle Bob had a 12-step plan for every hobby?" You can even organize a "take one home" system—guests can draw straws or play rock-paper-scissors for the right to claim a prized possession.

Just imagine the laughs as friends reminisce about the time Uncle Larry wore that outrageous Hawaiian shirt to Thanksgiving—or the bewilderment over why Aunt June had 27 miniature garden gnomes. In the end, gifting personal items can turn a somber occasion into a delightful scavenger hunt, ensuring that your loved ones leave with a piece of you—and maybe a goofy story or two to share for years to come!

_____
_____
_____
_____
_____
_____

Release

The Great Send-Off: Because Balloons Are So Last Year!

Many celebrations involve a symbolic send-off, and while balloon releases might seem like a classic move, let's be honest: they're about as eco-friendly as a plastic fork at a barbecue. So why not get creative and choose a send-off that won't make Mother Nature weep?

Consider some alternatives that are just as beautiful but far less harmful! You could release butterflies and let them flutter away like your hopes and dreams on a Monday morning. Doves are always a classy touch—who doesn't love a bird that looks like it just came from a spa day? Or how about bamboo lanterns? They're like candles, but you get to pretend you're on a magical Asian vacation while you release them!

And let's not forget the ultimate fun option: bubbles! Yes, bubbles! Imagine everyone at your celebration blowing bubbles into the air while giggling like kids. It's whimsical, it's lighthearted, and it's guaranteed to bring out the inner child in everyone—plus, they're way less likely to get stuck in a tree!

Feeling a bit more adventurous? How about having each guest write a goodbye message and toss it into a bonfire during your ceremony? Just picture the sight of messages rising up in smoke while everyone watches. "Bye-bye, cruel world!" and "I still can't believe you thought pineapple belonged on pizza!" will make for some memorable moments.

So skip the balloons, and let your send-off be as unique as you were! Whether it's butterflies, bubbles, or bonfire notes, it's time to create a send-off that's not only beautiful but also hilarious—and completely free of guilt!

Do you want a release? What kind of release would you like to have?

_____

_____

_____

_____

In Lieu of flowers 🌱

Do you have a favorite charity? _____

Are you passionate about a cause? _____

_____

"In Lieu of Flowers" – Think Outside the Bouquet

Flowers are lovely, but let's be honest—they wilt faster than your cousin can eat through the post-funeral buffet. Instead of the usual floral arrangements, why not get creative with how people can honor your memory? Here are some offbeat and meaningful ideas for donations in your name:

- **Support Your Passions:** Loved vintage bowling shirts? Have people donate to a retro fashion museum. Obsessed with cats? Set up a fund for the local animal shelter to name a room after you—preferably the one with the best snacks.

- **Random Acts of Kindness:** Ask folks to pay it forward—buy a stranger's coffee, leave a big tip, or pay for the person behind them in the drive-thru. Just imagine the ripple effect of all that good karma!

- **Scholarships for the Quirky:** Create a scholarship for aspiring accordion players, amateur magicians, or folks who can recite all 50 state capitals in alphabetical order. Make it specific, fun, and oh-so-you.

- **Sponsor an Experience:** Instead of buying roses, have people fund a rollercoaster ride day for underprivileged kids or a skydiving trip for your thrill-seeking niece.

- **Green Your Legacy:** Request donations for planting trees, cleaning up parks, or protecting bees. Bonus points if they plant a forest in your name and call it something punny, like "Your Lasting Grove."

- **Fund a Quirky Project**: Loved local theater? Ask for donations to support productions. Passionate about knitting? Help fund a community project to make scarves for the homeless. Want your sense of humor to live on? Fund a comedy class or stand-up night.

- **Sponsor a Playlist:** Ask friends to donate to a cause while creating a playlist of songs that remind them of you. Bonus points if it's a mix of meaningful ballads and guilty-pleasure hits.

- **Food for Thought:** Have donations go to a local food bank or soup kitchen. Even better, start a tradition where everyone shares a meal in your honor—tacos, anyone?

- **Library Love:** Were you a bookworm? Request donations for a local library, literacy program, or even to fund a little free library stocked with your favorite reads.

- **Artistic Legacy:** Fund public art projects, community murals, or a class for aspiring artists. Imagine your name attached to a splash of color downtown!

- **Adopt a Highway (or Bench):** Leave a mark by sprucing up a stretch of road or dedicating a park bench in your name. Your loved ones will think of you every time they sit for a snack or dodge a pothole.

- **Tech Forward:** Request donations to provide laptops, tablets, or internet access for students or seniors. It's a gift that connects people—just like you always did.

- **Support Weird Hobbies:** Loved model trains? Vintage typewriters? Collectible spoons? Start a fund to support niche museums or hobby clubs. It's wonderfully specific and 100% memorable.

- **Charity Challenges:** Encourage loved ones to participate in a charity run, walk, or polar plunge in your memory. Bonus if you request they wear something ridiculous like neon tutus or banana costumes.

- **Celebrate Science:** Was STEM your jam? Fund a research project, donate to a science museum, or help send kids to space camp. You'll be shooting for the stars, literally.

- **Sponsor Travel:** Loved adventure? Set up a fund to send someone on a trip they'd never take otherwise. Whether it's Paris, Peru, or the closest beach, you'll be their passport to joy.

- **Game On:** Were you into sports or games? Ask people to donate to buy equipment for a local youth team or start a chess club. If you were a lifelong fan, maybe even fund a stadium seat with your name on it.

- **Support Animal Rescues:** In addition to shelters, consider something specific like sponsoring therapy animals, service dog training, or a farm animal sanctuary. "In honor of [Your Name], defender of ducks!" has a nice ring to it.

- **Local Legends Fund:** Encourage donations to quirky local causes like the town museum, historical society, or annual pancake breakfast. Keep your community spirit alive and kicking.

- **Bail Someone Out (Literally):** No, not your cousin. Set up a fund for organizations that help pay off student loans, medical debt, or other financial burdens for those in need.

These ideas are as diverse and interesting as life itself. Whether they make people laugh, cry, or go, "That's so *them!*" they'll keep your legacy alive in the best ways possible.

MEMORIALS AND COMMEMORATIONS

 There are countless ways to celebrate and honor our loved ones after they've passed—get creative! If they had a hobby or favorite pastime, turn it into a party with purpose. Was golf their thing? Host a golf outing, and don't worry if no one knows how to play—mini-golf works too. Big fan of sports? Organize a baseball game, even if it's just a bunch of people fumbling in the backyard. Bowling? Go wild with team names like "Rolling in Their Memory."

Maybe your loved one loved trivia or karaoke—combine the two for an unforgettable night where every wrong answer or off-key note gets a laugh. Or, throw a movie or bingo night, because nothing says "I miss you" like yelling "Bingo!" at the top of your lungs.

Did they enjoy giving back? Gather the troops for a day of cleaning up parks, feeding the homeless, or holding a yard sale where the proceeds go to their favorite charity. Bonus points if the yard sale includes their questionable taste in knick-knacks.

On their birthday, throw a party! Share stories, flip through photos, or serve their favorite foods (yes, even if that means Jell-O with fruit in it). Or try something unique, like planting a tree in their honor or doing a group hike at their favorite spot. Light up some sky lanterns, hold a backyard bonfire, or even organize a group paint night where everyone creates something inspired by them.

Are you a music lover? Then why not crank up the celebration with karaoke! Whether its heartfelt ballads or hilariously off-key renditions of "Don't Stop Believin'," it's guaranteed to be a hit. Not a singer? No problem! Let guests grab the mic to share their favorite story or memory—it's like karaoke for talkers. Who wouldn't want to hear Aunt Linda recount that family vacation gone wrong in front of a live audience? So, what do you think? Are we singing, storytelling, or just laughing at whoever gets brave enough to grab the mic first?

And whatever you decide to do, this is a perfect excuse to share stories, photos, and their favorite foods (even if their favorite was something strange, like sardines on toast). Celebrate big, laugh hard, and let their memory shine.

The following questions are to encourage you to think about your life now. Do not be modest or shy when answering. This is part of the story of how you lived, your hopes, dreams, personality. Help those you leave behind to understand you, your struggles, and the things that brought you joy. Let's have some fun with this! These questions are here to make you think about *you*—your quirks, your awesomeness, and your one-of-a-kind life. Don't hold back; this isn't the time to be modest or shy. Flex a little! This is your chance to leave behind the ultimate highlight reel: your hopes, dreams, personality, triumphs, and even those "facepalm" moments that make you, *you*. Help your future audience—friends, family, and maybe a nosy archaeologist—understand what made your life so amazing, messy, and totally worth it.

What song defines you?

What do you think is the difference between knowledge and wisdom?

What advice have you received that has stuck with you? Who was it from?

What type of people bring you down?

What type of people inspire you?

What would you want your children or next of kin to know if you were to die tomorrow?

Write down one thing you hope to have added to humanity:

What ignites you? (What makes you happy, sparks your flow or makes you lose track of time?

What feeds your soul? (What gives you goosebumps, leaves you speechless, or makes life worth living?)

Aside from romantic love, have you loved enough?

What 3 things do you feel are most important in life?

If you have a terminal illness at the end of your life, where do you prefer to spend your last days? (Remain at home or go to a controlled medical environment or nursing home?)

What is on your bucket list? What do you want to do, experience, or accomplish before you die?

What do you love doing that you want to do more of?

What worries you most?

What regrets do you have? Can they be rectified?

NOTES:_____

_____
_____
_____
_____
_____
_____
_____
_____
_____
_____
_____
_____
_____
_____
_____
_____
_____
_____
_____

Finally:

Copy this information. Store one in a secure location with your Advance Directives, Will, Legal papers, etc. and give a copy to someone you trust to carry out your wishes. **After you have completed this book, keep it with your important end-of-life papers.**

We are gathered here today to discuss our own demise, or rather, what happens after we die. Although this is a lighthearted book, it is a serious and important discussion to have with ourselves and our loved ones. Let's talk about the important documents everyone should have, ideally while they are healthy. Please take some time to review this page and have serious conversations at an **appropriate and a private time** with your loved ones.

Advanced Directives

Understanding Advanced Directives in the United States and Beyond

What are Advanced Directives?

An Advanced Directive is a legal document that communicates your healthcare preferences if you become unable to make decisions for yourself. It ensures that your wishes about medical treatment are respected, providing guidance to family members and healthcare providers. Advanced Directives typically include two main components: Along with the two most common directives below, we also should consider organ/tissue donation and DNR orders as Advance Directives.

Medical (or Healthcare) Power of Attorney (might be known as agent, proxy, representative, or surrogate depending on where you reside.) This document designates a person (aka proxy) that you elect to make healthcare decisions for you ONLY if you are unable to communicate your wishes on your own. Specifies your preferences for life-sustaining treatments, such as mechanical ventilation, resuscitation, or artificial nutrition. This is different from a Financial Power of Attorney.

Living Will

This document informs your medical team how you wish to receive medical care and treatments if you are unable to make these decisions on your own.

Requirements in the United States:
It must be in writing.
The individual must be of sound mind and typically at least 18 years old.
Signatures of the individual and witnesses (or notarization) are required.
Some states have additional requirements for specific forms or registry options.

Variation by State:

Laws differ from state to state. For example, some states allow POLST (Physician Orders for Life-Sustaining Treatment) forms, which are medical orders that accompany Advanced Directives. Others have specific registries where documents can be stored for easy access by healthcare providers.

Notable Points:

Advanced Directives are not binding across state lines but are often honored. Regular updates are recommended to ensure preferences are current.

Other countries recognize the importance of planning ahead but may use different terms, formats, or legal frameworks. (Illustration purposes only, not legal information.) Here's a look at how some countries approach Advanced Directives:

Canada:

- Known as *Advance Care Planning*. Each province and territory has its own laws.
- **Requirements:**
    - Generally includes a written document expressing preferences (Living Will) and a designated proxy (Power of Attorney for Personal Care).
    - No national form; regulations vary significantly.
- Quebec, for instance, has strict laws requiring notarized documents for specific decisions like medical aid in dying.

United Kingdom:

- Known as *Advance Decision to Refuse Treatment (ADRT)* or *Advance Statement*.
- **Requirements:**
    - Must be in writing, signed, and witnessed for life-sustaining treatments.
    - Must specify treatments to be refused and under what circumstances.
    - Legal under the Mental Capacity Act of 2005.
- **Notable Point:** An Advance Decision cannot demand specific treatments, only refuse them.

41

Australia:

- Called *Advance Care Directives* (ACD).

- **Requirements:**

  o   Each state and territory has its own rules and forms.

  o   Generally includes both treatment preferences and the appointment of a medical decision-maker.

- States like Victoria recognize ACDs as legally binding, while others may treat them as advisory.

Germany:

- Known as *Patientenverfügung (Patient Directive)*.

- **Requirements:**

  o   Must be in writing and explicitly state treatment preferences.

  o   Highly specific, detailing treatments under various conditions (e.g., terminal illness, coma).

  o   No age restriction, but the person must be of sound mind.

- Binding on doctors if it meets all legal criteria.

Japan:

- No national law mandates Advanced Directives, but voluntary programs and templates exist.

- Documents often focus on preferences for end-of-life care and appointing a healthcare proxy.

- Cultural preferences often lean toward family decision-making rather than formal documentation.

Netherlands:

- Advanced Directives include *euthanasia requests* in countries where euthanasia is legal.

  o   **Requirements:** Must be written and reviewed with a physician. Includes details on acceptable treatments and life-ending measures in terminal situations.

Why Advanced Directives Matter

Wherever you are, having an Advanced Directive ensures your medical preferences are respected and reduces stress for loved ones during difficult times. Legal frameworks vary, so it's important to understand local laws and update your directive if you move or your health changes. Consulting a healthcare provider or legal expert is often helpful when preparing these documents.

Advanced Directives are legal documents each of us should have. They are ONLY used if you cannot communicate your wishes and can be changed at any time if you can communicate your wishes. These documents help those left behind to stress less because the plan has been made to our person's preferences. There will not be any guessing or questioning about what they want.

These documents are called Directives because they help the dying person direct their medical team, friends, loved ones, and caregivers to their end-of-life wishes. While this can be created at any time, many people, unfortunately, wait until they are in the throes of death to start this conversation. At that time there is a lot of stress and sadness. Much of what all parties are feeling goes unmentioned.

Other important documents you should have before death are a legal Will (last will) and a Durable Power of Attorney for Finances. A will is a legal document created to state your intentions on how your estate will be managed, divided, or distributed. It also addressed children under 18 years of age and adult dependents.

A Durable Power of Attorney for Finances is a legal document naming someone to make financial decisions for you, but ONLY if you are unable to. This is different from a Medical Durable Power of Attorney.

Important Note: Some states in the U.S. do not require a will to be drawn up by an attorney. You usually DO need to be at least 18 years old and of sound mind. Get a Notary. You will need at least two witnesses. You may wish to contact an attorney if you think the will could be contested or if you wish to disinherit someone. You may want to retain a lawyer for peace of mind as well. CHECK WITH YOUR STATE OR LOCAL AGENCY FOR LEGAL REQUIREMENTS for requirements in your jurisdiction on Advance Directives as well as wills and Financial Durable Power of Attorney.

*This information is subject to change at any time and should not be used to make legal decisions. Please consult an attorney in your locality for up-to-date advice and counsel.

www.ingramcontent.com/pod-product-compliance
Lightning Source LLC
Chambersburg PA
CBHW060856270326
41934CB00003B/169